Soul Ties

An Inside Look

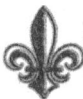

McDougal & Associates
Servants of Christ and Stewards of the
Mysteries of God

Soul Ties

An Inside Look

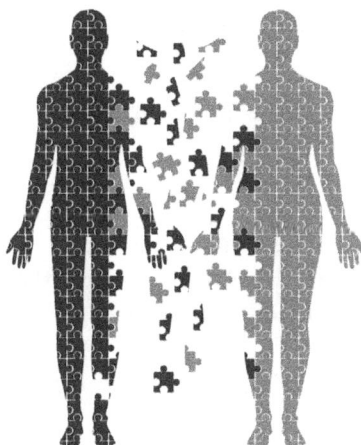

by

Jane P. McCoy

Cover image from Shutterstock.com

Published by:

McDougal & Associates
18896 Greenwell Springs Road
Greenwell Springs, LA 70739

www.ThePublishedWord.com

McDougal & Associates is an organization dedicated to the spreading of the Gospel of the Lord Jesus Christ to as many people as possible in the shortest time possible.

ISBN: 978-1-950398-24-9

Printed in the U.S., the U.K. and Australia
For Worldwide Distribution

Dedication

I dedicate this book to my grandsons (Jacory Perrault, Jayden Perrault, Jay E. Perrault and Jacoby Perrault) and granddaughters (Paradise M. Brown and Armani P. Moore). May God always be first in your lives, as He continues to build you up and bless you with all His promises. Thanks for being a major part of my life. You make my heart sing, and I am proud.

With much love,
Your Grandmother Jane

Contents

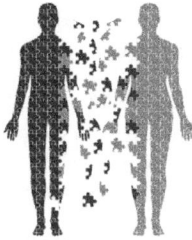

Introduction

Soul ties is a subject that can be confusing to many and on many different levels as well. I know this because for a long time I didn't understand the biblical definition of soul ties myself. During my research, the Lord has given me a more clear understanding, so I desire to share what I have learned with others.

Soul ties is a phrase we use to refer to a spiritual connection between two people or between a person and an animal or thing. What I didn't know was that there are different types of soul ties. This ignorance left me uninformed to the seriousness of soul ties. Being connected to the wrong person or things comes with ramifications. Every person's life is deeply affected by soul ties, whether those soul ties are good or evil.

Soul ties can be formed in one of several ways. Good soul ties are formed between husband and wife through their sexual union and consistent fellowship. Bad soul ties are formed between the participants of any illicit sex act. Good soul ties are formed between parents and their children through the normal nurturing process. Bad soul ties are formed when parents are abusive, neglectful or are unloving. Good soul ties can also be formed through close friendships and alliances. These can also be in business. Bad soul ties are formed through alliances with the wrong people. God has said in His Word:

> *Be ye not unequally yoked together with unbelievers: for what fellowship hath righteousness with unrighteousness? and what communion hath light with darkness? And what concord hath Christ with Belial? or what part hath he that believeth with an infidel? And what agreement hath the temple of God with idols? for ye are the temple of the living God; as God hath said, I will dwell in them, and walk in them; and I will be their God, and they shall be my people. Wherefore come out from among them, and be ye separate, saith the Lord, and touch not the unclean thing; and I will receive you. And will*

Introduction

*be a Father unto you, and ye shall be my sons
and daughters, saith the Lord Almighty.*

2 Corinthians 6:14-18

Many in society today (and also in the Body of
Christ) suffer from the consequences of wrong
soul ties and don't even know it. But living a
broken, detached and incomplete life is not
what God has for His children. Jesus Christ
died that we could live a fulfilled life, a life of
meaning, a life of purpose and a life progres-
sively moving forward.

Therefore, I am authoring this book to help
others. I pray that these writings, under the
anointing of the Holy Spirit, will bring you
wisdom, knowledge and understanding con-
cerning this important subject and how it can
impact the lives of God's people.

I pray for your liberty as you address the
negative soul ties in your life that you may have
previously overlooked or ignored. Now is the
time for reckoning. May God grant you grace
to be set free.

*In Jesus' name,
Amen!*

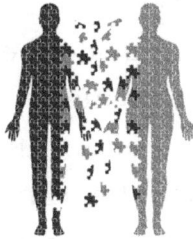

What Is a Soul Tie?

If you have ever ended a relationship, whether it was a business relationship or personal relationship, and felt you somehow could not get past it, a soul tie was definitely present, and needs to be broken. A soul tie is a covenant in which two souls become entwined. There are righteous soul ties, and there are demonic soul ties.

When there is a soul tie, we become *"one flesh,"* according to the Bible. Two souls are united, joined or knit together. Soul ties may be invisible, but they are real. They can be between humans and animals, either alive or already passed. Examples of soul ties between live humans would be husband and wife, a man and a whore, a woman and a male prostitute, two men or two women. Soul ties between the living and the dead can include the inability of a surviving spouse to give up the dead partner or an undue influence of the dead upon the living. Soul ties can also be between a human, male or female, and a beast.

The Bible doesn't use the term *soul ties*, but it does talk about souls being knit together or *"the twain shall become one flesh"* in the Spirit realm. Even though soul ties are spiritual (and thus, unseen), they must not be underestimated. Since there are godly soul ties, and there are demonic soul ties, we must know the difference or suffer the consequences.

Have you been married and divorced or separated? Has your spouse died? If so, you may still have a soul tie with that person that needs to be broken (unless, of course, you plan to reunite with a living spouse after a temporary separation). Soul ties can leave an individual in broken pieces, unable to function in the complete scope of their purpose.

John 2:12, AMPC

> *When they had all had enough, He said to His disciples, Gather up now the fragments (the*

broken pieces that are left over), so that nothing may be lost and wasted.

Fragment can be defined as "a part broken off, detached, or incomplete." If you had sex outside of marriage, committed adultery, or have been divorced or separated, you must break the soul ties you formed with that person through sex. Otherwise, it may be impossible for you to live the richest life possible. Instead, you may remain broken, detached and incomplete.

Marriage As a Covenant Relationship

God Himself founded marriage, and He intended it to be a covenant relationship. This is important to understand, for it helps us to better understand the issue of soul ties. *The Legal Dictionary* states, "A biblical marriage is a legally sanctioned contract between a man and a woman. Entering a marriage contract changes the legal status of both parties, giving husband and wife new rights and obligations. Public policy is strongly in favor of marriage based on the belief that it preserves the family unit."[1]

1. https://legaldictionary.thefreedictionary.com/marriage

More importantly, marriage is an agreement before God, a covenant if you will, and every covenant has three elements. There are the PROMISES, what you will receive from the covenant. There are the AGREEMENTS, what is expected from each person who enters into the covenant. And there are the CONDITIONS, what each one must do in order to receive the fullest benefits of the covenant. Your walk with God is a covenant agreement, and so is your marriage.

The Promises

On their wedding day, a couple repeats a series of vows to publicly affirm—before God, before a minister and before other witnesses—their lifelong commitment to each other.

The Agreement

After the vows are repeated, the minister then asks each one some serious questions. Addressing them by name so that there can be no mistake about who is making this agreement, he asks, "Do you … ?" and the proper response is always, "I do." Those are strong

English words and they affirm the agreement. Once the couple agrees to the promises, then the marriage covenant is legally sealed in the eyes of God, the minister and the witnesses, and the minister pronounces them to be man and wife.

The Conditions

While love should be unconditional, the marriage vows come with spiritual conditions. One of the most important condition is faithfulness to your marriage partner. When a partner becomes unfaithful by committing adultery, the marriage vows are broken and heartache follows. Some marriages can be restored through humility and repentance, but far too often the act of adultery causes the innocent spouse to be crushed in spirit, which leads to separation and, ultimately, to divorce.

How sad! God hates divorce (see Malachi 2:16), and we should too, for it is destructive to everyone involved (especially innocent children), and it dishonors God. The epidemic of divorce and remarriage in our modern society have led to a an epidemic of soul ties and their often destructive consequences.

What Is Consummating a Marriage?

Consummation of Marriage is a legal term that refers "to the first time the husband and wife co-habit together or engage in sexual intercourse after the ceremony of marriage has been performed. Under canon law, a refusal to consummate the marriage may be grounds for an annulment or for divorce."[2]

Consummating the marriage was what God had in mind when He instituted marriage in the first place:

Genesis 2:24

Therefore, shall a man leave his father and his mother, and shall cleave unto his wife: and they shall be one flesh.

This concept was repeated in the New Testament to show us its eternal aspect:

Ephesians 5:31

For this cause shall a man leave his father and mother, and shall be joined unto his wife, and they two shall be one flesh.

2. definitions.uslegal.com/c/consummation-of-marriage/

What Is a Soul Tie?

That the two become *"one flesh"* is based upon a biblical and godly covenant, alliance, or allegiance between the two of them, and *"one flesh"* was intended to and should involve a life-long bond (the covenant that God established) in all physical, emotional and spiritual matters. This is a unique bond that God established for our benefit. Unfortunately, when the seriousness of marriage is not respected, what follows is a lot of hurt and confusion and the lingering consequences of soul ties.

Let us define some of these words and phrases as used in the Holy Bible.

One (H259, *ekh-awd'*) "properly united, that is, one; or (as an ordinal) first: a, alike, alone, a certain (dail-)ly, each (one)," from (H258, *aw-khad'*) "to unify, that is, (figuratively) collect (one's thoughts): go one way or other."

Flesh (H1320, *baw-sawr'*) "flesh, by extension body, person, kin, kind, nakedness, self, skin."

Joined (G4347, *proskollao*) "to glue to, that is, (figuratively) to adhere; cleave, join (self)."

Soul Ties: An Inside Look

Every human being is composed of spirit, soul and body:

1 Thessalonians 5:23

And the very God of peace sanctify you wholly; and I pray God your whole spirit and soul and body be preserved blameless unto the coming of our Lord Jesus Christ.

Soul (G5590, *psyche*) "breath, that is, (by implication), spirit." Your soul is the part of you that consists of your mind, character, thoughts, and feelings, your will and your emotions.

Ties, "a thing that unites or links people." Some examples are contracts, covenants, relationships, allegiances, oaths, alliances, etc. These words and their meanings show us how soul ties bind individuals to each other in the mind (*psyche'*, e.g. the spirit realm).

Why do we have so many problems in this area today? It is because we partake of the promise of marriage without accepting the responsibilities of marriage. The result is that we find ourselves under a curse instead of the blessing God intended.

Covenant and Responsibilities

We must always lean on the Word of God to validate our belief system, and we must use the Scriptures to prove our thoughts. The Bible makes itself clear, and therein, we can discern good from evil.

A covenant involves conditions, agreements and outcomes. The word *covenant* itself can be defined as "a usually formal, solemn and binding agreement: compact." The first covenant noted in the Bible was the covenant between God and man. It was called the Edenic Covenant (see Genesis 2:15-17). This covenant required certain things of Adam:

- To propagate the human race
- To subdue the earth for mankind
- To have dominion over the animal creation
- To care for the garden and eat of its fruits and herbs and
- To abstain from eating of one tree, the tree of the knowledge of good and evil, on penalty of death for disobedience.

It was only after God had made this agreement with Adam that He instituted the first marriage. The marriage He instituted was a union between a man and a woman, but it had a third party. That third party was God Himself. He was to be the Arbiter of the marriage and its Guide. The man and the woman, for their part, vowed to comply righteously with their God-given covenant.

Sex in marriage, as God envisioned it, had two purposes: 1). It was for the propagation of the human race, but 2). It was also the glue that would hold the marriage together. Of all of the members of the animal kingdom, sex between humans is unique. With the other animals, it is solely for procreation, and very often the male and female animals then part and go their separate ways. God made human sexuality so enjoyable that it would keep the man and the woman in a close-knit family setting to raise their young together and be a blessing to each other.

So one responsibility of a man and his wife is propagation. What is propagation?

To *propagate* means "1. to cause to continue or increase by sexual or asexual reproduction, 2.

to pass along to offspring, 3. to cause to spread out and affect a greater number or greater area: extend." God has proven through His Word that He supplies what is needed to fulfill what is required of us. For righteous reproduction, we must first be in the covenant relationship of marriage.

God said:

1 Corinthians 7:2

Nevertheless, to avoid fornication, let every man have his own wife, and let every woman have her own husband.

Our bodies are God's temple and were not meant for indiscriminate sex:

1 Corinthians 6:17-18

But he that is joined unto the Lord is one spirit. Flee fornication. Every sin that a man doeth is without the body; but he that committeth fornication sinneth against his own body.

The womb of a woman is God's treasure chest:

Psalm 127:3

> *Lo, children are an heritage of the Lord: and the fruit of the womb is his reward.*

In this next scripture passage, notice how concerned God is with our marriage covenant:

Malachi 2:13-16

> *And this have ye done again, covering the altar of the Lord with tears, with weeping, and with crying out, insomuch that he regardeth not the offering any more, or receiveth it with good will at your hand. Yet ye say, Wherefore? Because the Lord hath been witness between thee and the wife of thy youth, against whom thou hast dealt treacherously: yet is she thy companion, and the wife of thy covenant. And did not he make one? Yet had he the residue of the spirit. And wherefore one? That he might seek a godly seed. Therefore take heed to your spirit, and let none deal treacherously against the wife of his youth. For the Lord, the God of Israel, saith that he hateth putting away: for one covereth violence with his garment, saith the Lord of hosts: therefore take heed to your spirit, that ye deal not treacherously.*

Yes, a marriage, in the eyes of the Lord, is between a man and a woman, and it is for the purpose of producing a godly seed.

Wife (H802, *ishshah*) "a woman, a wife (woman married to a man)."

Husband (H376, *iysh*) "a man as an individual or a male person."

So, first, the Lord created sex between the married man and woman to propagate the earth. Let's stop here to say that this casts a spotlight on certain sexual practices as being deviant. Any mechanical means of sexual release would not result in reproduction. The use of sex tools and other foreign objects might be socially accepted, but they cannot be accepted by God. And He is the one who counts.

His command to the man and woman was this:

Genesis 1:28
> *And God blessed them, and God said unto them, Be fruitful, and multiply, and replenish the earth.*

What did God mean? He meant for them to reproduce, to propagate the human species, and oral and anal sex (sodomy) cannot fulfill this requirement. Sodomy is a perversion that leaves one with ungodly soul ties that must be broken. That spirit must be cast out.

The second purpose for sex, serving as the glue that would hold the marriage together, also presents a problem. God made sex so enjoyable that carnal men use it in many perverted ways, outside of God's intention and against His clearly defined guidelines for its use. This brings a curse.

Remember what God said:

Hosea 4:6

My people are destroyed for lack of knowledge: because thou hast rejected knowledge, I will also reject thee, that thou shalt be no priest to me: seeing thou hast forgotten the law of thy God, I will also forget thy children.

Now you know, and a lack of knowledge can only lead to captivity and ruin.

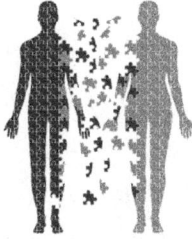

– 2 –

Demonic Soul Ties

Demonic soul ties are soul ties developed through unrighteous acts. These would include:

Soul Ties formed through Fornication

An unrighteous soul tie happens when some-one has sex outside of the marriage covenant. Fornication and adultery are acts outside of a godly marriage union. Fornication would include sex between men and women before marriage, even if the consenting adults get married afterward. A soul tie is formed immediately upon their sexual union.

1 Corinthians 6:18
> *Flee fornication. Every sin that a man doeth is*

*without the body; but he that committeth forni-
cation sinneth against his own body.*

Fornication (G4202, *porneia*) "harlotry, including adultery and incest; figuratively, idolatry"
(from G4203, *porneuo*) "to act the harlot, that
is, (literally) indulge unlawful lust (of either
sex)," (from G4204) "a strumpet; figuratively
an idolater; harlot, whore."

Soul Ties formed through Adultery

Adultery is an ungodly sexual act between a
married person and someone who is not their
legitimate mate. God said:

Exodus 20:14
Thou shalt not commit adultery.

Adultery can also be defined as "fornication."
If a man or woman has sex outside of marriage with another, a soul tie is formed with
that person. Then, when that married person
goes to bed with their true mate, it is as if they
were bringing the other person in with them.

This causes problems with intimacy and sexual performance. Why? Because there are always other persons coming between them in their marriage and love life. What God has joined together must not be separated:

Matthew 19:6

> *Wherefore they are no more twain, but one flesh. What therefore God hath joined together, let not man put asunder.*

Let us look at the meanings of these words:

Twain (G1417) "duo; two."

Hath joined together (G4801, *suzeugnumi*) "to yoke together, that is (figuratively) conjoin (in marriage)" from (G4862) "sun; denoting union; with or together; association, companionship."

Put asunder (G5569; chorizo) "to place room between, that is, part; reflexively, to go away; depart, put asunder, separate."

The continued health of a marriage requires, first, the acknowledgement of any sin that can harm it. Then, there must be repentance for that sin and renunciation of that sin. And, finally, you must break that ungodly soul tie.

Soul Ties formed through Homosexuality

Homosexuality forms soul ties between men, just as Lesbianism forms soul ties between women. They have united their souls through the sexual acts of sodomy and/or oral sex. God said they have become knit together. In Old Testament times, there was a severe punishment for this act of rebellion against God:

Leviticus 20:13

If a man also lie with mankind, as he lieth with a woman, both of them have committed an abomination: they shall surely be put to death; their blood shall be upon them.

Thank God for what Jesus Christ has done for sinners. He has become our peace. Confess your faults, turn from your wicked works, and live. Jesus is the remedy for your sins.

Soul Ties formed through Bestiality

Way back in the beginning, as Adam named all the beasts God had created, there was not one of them fit to be his companion. No beast is equal to a human being. Then God said:

Genesis 2:18 and 20

> *And the LORD God said, It is not good that the man should be alone; I will make him an help meet for him.*
> *And Adam gave names to all cullle, and to the fowl of the air, and to every beast of the field; but for Adam there was not found an help meet for him.*

These passages confirm God's intentions. Every beast was to reproduce after its own kind, and, in the same way, humans were to reproduce with humans, a man and a woman.

Bestiality is a subject that is rarely addressed. Society ignores it, hoping it will just go away or take care of itself. But it won't. Bestiality is the sexual union between a man or woman and a beast. Even though this is an unlawful act in many states, it still happens, and when it does, an ungodly soul tie is formed.

God said:

Leviticus 18:23

Neither shalt thou lie with any beast to defile thyself therewith: neither shall any woman stand before a beast to lie down thereto: it is confusion.

Deuteronomy 27:21

Cursed be he that lieth with any manner of beast. And all the people shall say, Amen.

What can we do if we have been cursed in this way? Jesus Christ became a curse for us:

Galatians 3:13

Christ hath redeemed us from the curse of the law, being made a curse for us: for it is written, Cursed is every one that hangeth on a tree.

God provided a remedy for every curse, both those we have inherited and those we bring upon ourselves. Praise God for His great love for us.

God created man for woman, and woman for man, and the keeping of His sacred covenant to be fruitful and replenish the earth requires human to human and beast to beast interaction. Any manipulation of His Word to attempt to justify man's ungodly lusts will be judged by the sword of His mouth. He said:

1 Corinthians 6:9-10

> *Know ye not that the unrighteous shall not inherit the kingdom of God? Be not deceived: neither fornicators, nor idolaters, nor adulterers, nor effeminate, nor abusers of themselves with mankind, nor thieves, nor covetous, nor drunkards, nor revilers, nor extortioners, shall inherit the kingdom of God.*

Galatians 5:18

> *But if ye be led of the Spirit, ye are not under the law.*

Soul Ties formed through Masturbation

Masturbation is another means by which the people of God can come into soulish covenant with demonic foes. Satan uses the sex drive to trap as many as he can, especially Christians. Masturbation is a form of self-indulgence and self-love. It is strictly a selfish pleasure and produces doubt, condemnation and failure. Satan's lie is that it does not involve anyone else, so no one is harmed and, therefore, it is acceptable to God. That is not true.

The more times you engage in any deviant sexual activity, including masturbation, the more difficult it becomes to break the practice and the resulting soul ties. Being as persistent to resist the demons as the demons are persistent against you will put you in proper submission to God, and the devil will flee (see James 4:5-8).

Masturbation opens doors to other sex demons. These demons have been given names: Incubus and Succubus. The Christian community knows these two sex demons well, for they visit you while you sleep. Incubus is a male demon believed to have sexual intercourse with sleeping women, and Succubus is a female demon believed to have sexual intercourse with sleeping men.

Masturbation is never okay in any situation, and the soul ties that result from this ungodly practice must be broken.

Soul Ties Formed through Pornography

Sadly, pornography has become acceptable entertainment today in many homes around our nation and the world. Flourishing because of the proliferation of the internet, it is another means by which the people of God come into soulish covenant with demonic forces.

Pornography is a major threat to marriage, to the family and to society at large. It is not, as many believe, a private choice without public consequences. Pornography alters both sexual attitudes and behavior, undermining marriage. This, in turn, undermines the stability of the entire community. The use of pornography is a pathway to infidelity and divorce and is frequently a major factor in family disasters.

Whenever pornography is presented to the eyegate, the soulish man becomes susceptible to the entrance and operation of demons. What you see with your eyes opens the door to your heart. Then, once demons become occupants, they have legal rights to that temple ... unless and until that wicked alliance is broken. The participant has joined himself to another and is seeking sexual gratification by means contrary to the original covenant God made with Adam from the beginning: *"multiply and replenish the earth."*

Porn stars are now interfering with the marriage and have become the thing which separates the man and the woman. The two participants—the porn star and the customer—may never meet face to face, but the effect of this fantasy is detrimental to the marriage nevertheless. The participant becomes entangled by this ungodly relationship.

Couples affected by one spouse's addiction to pornography usually experience a loss of interest in sexual intercourse and good family relations. The spirits of fantasy lust, incubus, succubus and all other sex demons must be caste out and the devilish soul tie broken.

According to webroot.com, "The negative effects of pornography do not end after development. They can be just as harmful to families and marriages:

- According to the National Coalition for the Protection of Children and Families (2010), 47% of families in the United States reported that pornography is a problem in their home.
- Pornography use increases the marital infidelity rate by more than 300%.
- 40% of people identified as 'sex addicts' lose their spouses, 58% suffer considerable financial losses, and about 33% lose their jobs.
- 68% of divorce cases involve one party meeting a new paramour over the internet, while 56% involve one party having an 'obsessive interest' in pornographic websites."[3]

Soul Ties Formed through Wicked Alliances

Soul ties can also be formed through wicked alliances. This can occur in leadership or business settings. The Bible gives the example of Jehoshaphat, king of Judah. He was said to be a righteous king, and the Lord was with him:

3. https://www.webroot.com/us/en/resources/tips-articles/internet-pornography-by-the-numbers

2 Chronicles 17:3

> *And the LORD was with Jehoshaphat, because he walked in the first ways of his father David, and sought not unto Baalim.*

However, Jehoshaphat made a step in the wrong direction when he decided to make a marriage alliance. His son would marry the daughter of the wicked Queen Jezebel, wife of the infamous Ahab. Why would Jehoshaphat do something so foolish? Making an alliance with the wicked cannot lead to anything good.

2 Chronicles 18:1 and 3

> *Now Jehoshaphat had riches and honour in abundance and joined affinity with Ahab. And Ahab king of Israel said unto Jehoshaphat king of Judah, Wilt thou go with me to Ramothgilead? And he answered him, I am as thou art, and my people as thy people; and we will be with thee in the war.*

The righteous can never make an agreement with evil men or the wickedness they do. The Scriptures reveal this so clearly:

Amos 3:3

Can two walk together, except they be agreed?

It's a good question, and the answer is NO! Two cannot walk together unless they agree, and there is no agreement between good and bad:

2 Corinthians 6:14-18

Be ye not unequally yoked together with unbelievers: for what fellowship hath righteousness with unrighteousness? and what communion hath light with darkness? And what concord hath Christ with Belial? or what part hath he that believeth with an infidel? And what agreement hath the temple of God with idols? for ye are the temple of the living God; as God hath said, I will dwell in them, and walk in them; and I will be their God, and they shall be my people. Wherefore come out from among them, and be ye separate, saith the Lord, and touch not the unclean thing; and I will receive you. And will be a Father unto you, and ye shall be my sons and daughters, saith the Lord Almighty.

Soul Ties: An Inside Look

It is a risky business when we try to make an alliance of any kind with wicked people. That agreement may very well cause us to stray from God's presence at some point and go the way of unrighteousness. It's not worth the risk.

Very soon the Lord sent a prophet to rebuke Jehoshaphat, a seer named Jehu:

2 Chronicles 19:1-3

> *And Jehoshaphat the king of Judah returned to his house in peace to Jerusalem. And Jehu the son of Hanani the seer went out to meet him, and said to king Jehoshaphat, Shouldest thou help the ungodly, and love them that hate the LORD? therefore is wrath upon thee from before the LORD. Nevertheless there are good things found in thee, in that thou hast taken away the groves out of the land, and hast prepared thine heart to seek God.*

Bit it seems that Jehoshaphat did not learn his lesson. He made the same mistake again later:

2 Chronicles 20:35-37

> *Again, Jehoshaphat king of Judah, joined himself with the king of Israel, Ahaziah, and*

it displeased the LORD. And after this did Jehoshaphat king of Judah join himself with Ahaziah king of Israel, who did very wickedly: and he joined himself with him to make ships to go to Tarshish: and they made the ships in Eziongaber. Then Eliezer the son of Dodavah of Mareshah prophesied against Jehoshaphat, saying, because thou hast joined thyself with Ahaziah, the LORD hath broken thy works. And the ships were broken, that they were not able to go to Tarshish.

No matter who we happen to be, we cannot overwrite what God has said in His Word. An unrighteous soul tie can destroy your prosperity, wealth and increase, and, most importantly, can even cause the wrath of God to visit you. Be warned!

Soul Ties Formed through Sexual Lust

Judges 16 is about a ruler among the Israelites, one of their judges, named Samson. Samson had a weakness when it came to strange women, and that weakness became his downfall.

Soul Ties: An Inside Look

The people of Israel had a covenant relationship with the Lord that required them to marry within their own people. This would translate into Christians only marrying other Christians. Samson's first wife was a Philistine, and his next recorded encounter was with a harlot in Gaza. In the end, he met the infamous Delilah, and she betrayed him:

Judges 16:4

> *And it came to pass afterward, that he loved a woman in the valley of Sorek, whose name was Delilah.*

Samson was a very blessed and highly honored man. How sad that he chose to violate God's laws of sexual conduct! First, he married that Philistine woman, an unbeliever, and next, he had sex outside of marriage. In both of these cases, ungodly soul ties were formed. The saddest part may be that Samson didn't seem to realize how wrong these deeds were. Or did he not care for some reason?

Then Samson fell for Delilah and made her his second wife. But Delilah deceived him, taking a bribe of eleven hundred pieces of silver from the Philistine lords and delivering Samson into their hands. Samson's lust for strange women caused his downfall. He met a woman who had a demonic assignment, and he was blind to her treachery.

Anytime we violate the laws of God, there will be consequences. In this case, the consequences were tragic. Delilah had been on assignment for the enemy, and she delivered her man into their hands:

Judges 16:5

> *And the lords of the Philistines came up unto her, and said unto her, Entice him, and see wherein his great strength lieth, and by what means we may prevail against him, that we may bind him to afflict him; and we will give thee every one of us eleven hundred pieces of silver.*

Let us look at the details of this wicked assignment. It was:

- To entice Samson. *Entice* means "to lead on by exciting hope or desire, to allure and to tempt."

- To see where his great strength lay. Delilah was to examine his strength so the enemy kings could target and destroy it.
- To find out how the kings could prevail against Samson. *Prevail* means "to prove superior in strength and power."
- To bind him. One of the definitions of bind is "to imprison." Delilah did it so smoothly and apparently without remorse.
- To afflict him. *Afflict* translates as "to oppress, humble, be afflicted, and be bowed down."

The name Delilah can be interpreted as "delicate," but its root meaning is "to be brought low, to hang down and to be languid." *Languid* means "slow, lifeless, fatigued, weak, lacking in spirit and listless." As her name indicates, Delilah brought Samson low and weakened him. She did this by perverting his passion. In plain language, she seduced him, and the result was the he turned his passion away from God and focused it, instead, on worldly pleasures. Tragically, through her seductions, Delilah destroyed Samsons' destiny.[4]

4. Adapted from *Breaking the Threefold Demonic Cord, How to Discern and Defeat the Lies of Jezebel, Athaliah and Delilah* by

Demonic Soul Ties

In my previous books, I have made mention of the case of Linda and Joe, and as I began to write this book, I consulted again with Linda, this time about her experiences with soul ties. I was not disappointed. Linda had a remarkable and interesting story to tell regarding her bouts with ungodly soul ties. At this point, I would like to share her story.

Linda said that even after years of Joe's emotional, psychological and verbal abuse, once he was gone from her life, she had strong desires to have him back. An unseen force seemed to be pulling her back toward the very thing God had so graciously delivered her from. She felt physically ill and unable to cope without him, even though she had suffered stress-related illnesses while she was married to him.

Linda struggled with demonic soul ties that would not allow her to move on to new relationships after divorcing Joe. At first, she stated, she had no idea what the issue was until she became intimate with God again. As her relationship with God begun to grow, she was able to observe her behaviors and interactions

---

Sandie Freed (Grand Rapids, MI, Chosen Books: 2008)

much closer. They were not all healthy ones. She would sometimes daydream of herself and Joe in a very intimate manner—"fantasy lust." Joe had rejected and abandon her for another life, and yet she was fixated with him. Linda says, "I was not well. I needed to be delivered from my past. I needed to be set free from Joe and his hold. Somehow I needed to break this hold."

Linda shared very intimate details about her and Joe's sex life while they were married. Joe was not shy about trying different things sexually, and she went along for the ride. Both of them were guilty of having oral sex quiet frequently. Joe watched pornography and had extra marital affairs. In the end, Linda was convinced that she was wrestling with the spirit of perversion, which came in through Joe and his inordinate affections. He was a fornicator and an adulterer (see Colossians 3:5).

Because Joe had engaged in extra marital affairs and had also engaged in sexual relationships before their marriage, the soul ties were there, and they followed him. He was left fragmented, broken, and never coming to satisfaction with his life.

In a very real sense, Linda slept with every woman Joe had ever slept with, including the porn stars. Not only did she sleep with them; she became joined to them in the spirit realm, just as the Scriptures shows us. Whatever issues these people had became Joe's issues and, therefore, Linda's issues. Imagine trying to live a life of unknown identity, expecting to be fruitful, complete and restored. First, those soul ties had to be broken, and every fragment of Linda's soul would have to be recovered.

Since Linda has recovered, she has prayed for Joe's recovery. Soul ties bind your will, emotions and intellect (mind—*psyche'*).

Romans 7:25

> *I thank God through Jesus Christ our Lord. So then with the mind I myself serve the law of God; but with the flesh the law of sin.*

After a time, Linda was finally set free. It came about from walking through her deliverance, which included breaking those ungodly soul ties. Now, she is careful what she looks at and what she listens to. Her freedom is too important to lose again. She is so grateful to God for setting her free.

Soul Ties Formed through Witchcraft

Witchcraft can be defined as "the attempt to exercise control over others for personal gain." You don't have to be a witch or warlock to practice witchcraft.

A pastor or leader who tries to control his flock or group is practicing witchcraft. They may demand that their people disassociate themselves from others, except when they are present to monitor behaviors and interactions. Witchcraft is present when leaders use assigned positions and titles as a means to get others to become part of the movement. Witchcraft is present when the leader fails to speak truth for fear of losing control of the group. Witchcraft is present when others are motivated to do things under an atmosphere of fear and intimidation.

Soul ties are formed with those to whom we submit our wills. They can be formed with leaders of a church, as well as with any one in the occult that we go to for help. A dictatorial pastor can form soul ties with his congregation. Church leaders are cursed when they try to take the place of God in our lives, and a congregation is cursed when it follows man and not God.

We have no right to control others. God gives us a free will, and even He will not try to control us. Therefore, we enter into agreement with Satan and his demons when we attempt to control others and are guilty of practicing witchcraft.

Joe used his abusive behaviors to control Linda in public. He understood that she was well known, educated and proper, and she would do anything to keep him from showing out in front of others. He often presumed (in his mind) and made fun of Linda's inability (as he saw it) to support and care for herself when he would leave her. This caused him to often make threatening statements about leaving and not looking back.

According to Linda, none of those statements frightened her. They just made her wonder why Joe even bothered to call her his "wife." He was controlling and manipulating, and, according to Linda, always had a motive for whatever he did for her. That is a perfect picture of witchcraft being exercised between a husband and wife.

Linda's deliverance included breaking ungodly soul ties, breaking the power of witchcraft over her life and casting out demonic spirits that had come in through perverted sex acts.

Thank God, today she is free, and you can be too!

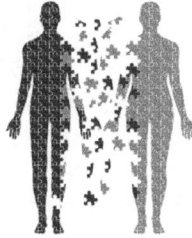

— 3 —

Soul Ties Between Parents and Their Children

Between parents and their children, there are both healthy and unhealthy soul ties that can be formed:

Healthy Soul Ties

When a child is born, a very normal spiritual bond, or soul tie, begins to be formed. Parents express their love for their child in many ways. When a healthy soul tie is formed, it ministers love and security to that child throughout life. The soul tie between parent and child stabilizes a child's personality. A healthy soul tie will support a child throughout life, and they will understand and have respect for healthy boundaries.

Unhealthy Soul Ties

An unhealthy soul tie is formed when parents allow the child to assume a role of authority in the home. This can happen for various reasons. It could be because of the death of one parent, a divorce, a lack of parenting or a debilitating illness. God's ordained order for the home is Christ as the head, then the husband, then the wife and only then the children.

Ephesians 5:23

For the husband is the head of the wife, even as Christ is the head of the church: and he is the saviour of the body.

Anything outside of the ordained precepts of God for the family is considered an act of disobedience and will always hinder the flow of blessings. Today, more then ever before, we have single-parent families for many reasons. The statistics are startling.

Soul Ties Between Parents and Their Children

According to U.S. Census data from 2015 (published in 2018), there are approximately 13.7 million single parents in the United States today, and those parents are responsible for raising 22.4 million children. This number represents approximately 27 % of children under the age of 21 in the U.S. today. According to Census data, approximately 80.4 % of custodial parents are mothers, and only 19.6 % of custodial parents (approximately 1 in 5) are fathers.[5]

An unhealthy soul tie is formed between the parent and child when the parents places a child in a role other than what is meant for the child. For example, some parent place a son in the role of "the man of the house," or a daughter as "the woman of the house." With these roles, go many God-given responsibilities that children are incapable of performing, and it is cruel to expect them to.

Tragically, some parents are amused by their own selfish and reckless behaviors. This reveals that they do not love their child as they should. Assigning anyone to a role they are not qualified for nor capable of fulfilling is not

5. www.verywellfamily.com; U.S. Census Bureau. Custodial Mothers and Fathers and their child support."

only irresponsible; it is also cruel and foolish because:

- First, that child is being placed in a position that is against his or her will.
- Second, the child cannot comprehend the scope of the duties and responsibilities inherent in that role.
- Third, that child cannot fulfill those duties, so he or she is being set up for failure.
- Fourth, the child is being forced to relinquish his or her rights as a child and assume an adult role given to him or her for someone else's personal gain.

If a parent does this, it is for one or more of the following reasons: manipulation, fear, ignorance, a sense of insecurity, lack of provision and/or protection. This unhealthy soul tie must be broken if both the child and parent are to be set free from spiritual contamination and spiritual bondage. If this tie is not broken, the child will become angry, controlling, dominating, manipulating and obsessed with any outside relationship the parent attempts to build. Because the child has been given illegitimate dominion over the home and the lives of those in the home, he or she feels threatened by any newcomer. A newcomer is seen as a threat to unseat the child from his or her position or reign.

Therefore, if and when a parent decides to remarry before this maze is worked out, the child will forever be the person separating the union of the parent and the new spouse. That union will never really take place in the spirit, because someone is always coming between the two of them.

Therefore, in order for both the child and the parent to build healthy relationships, this unhealthy soul tie must be broken. In order for the child to live a happy, productive and fulfilled life, he or she must be released from the role of fictitious husband or surrogate mother.

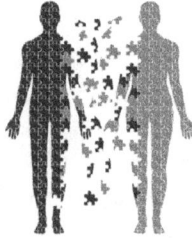

– 4 –

Righteous Soul Ties

So, as believers in Christ, we know what to avoid. Now, instead of focusing on the negative, we need to focus on the positive—righteous soul ties and how they are formed. I want to focus here on marriage and close friendships.

Soul Ties Formed through Marriage

God Himself instituted marriage,

Genesis 2:18 and 22-24

> *And the LORD God said, It is not good that the man should be alone; I will make him an help meet for him. And the LORD God caused a deep sleep to fall upon Adam, and he slept: and he took one of his ribs, and closed up the*

flesh instead thereof; and the rib, which the LORD God had taken from man, made he a woman, and brought her unto the man. And Adam said, This is now bone of my bones, and flesh of my flesh: she shall be called Woman, because she was taken out of Man. Therefore shall a man leave his father and his mother, and shall cleave unto his wife: and they shall be one flesh.

To prevent fornication, let each man and each woman have their own righteous partner by entering into a covenant or union in marriage:

1 Corinthians 7:2

Nevertheless, to avoid fornication, let every man have his own wife, and let every woman have her own husband.

The two, the man and the woman, are to be bound together in holy matrimony and become inseparable. What God has joined together, no man has a right to separate or put a space between. Marriage partners become knitted together in their souls to achieve the covenant purpose, propagation. In this way, a marriage bed is undefiled.

Hebrews 13:4

Marriage is honourable in all, and the bed undefiled: but whoremongers and adulterers God will judge.

Soul Ties Formed through Close Friendships

Soul ties can also be developed through close friendships. For instance, David had a soul tie with Jonathan, the son of King Saul.

Before David became king of Israel, he served as Saul's armorbearer, and during that time, he became close friends with Jonathan. In time, Saul became jealous of David and turned against him, but even then Jonathan remained a faithful friend.

Because of Saul's anger, David often had to flee for his life, but Jonathan kept him informed of his father's plans.

1 Samuel 18:1 and 3

And it came to pass, when he had made an end

of speaking unto Saul, that the soul of Jonathan was knit with the soul of David, and Jonathan loved him as his own soul.

Then Jonathan and David made a covenant, because he loved him as his own soul.

Let us define the word *knit:* (H7194, *kaw-shar'*) "to bind, league together, conspire." In other words, Jonathan made a legally binding agreement with David before the Lord. Later, Jonathan renewed his covenant with David. This demonstrates that both parties understood the importance of covenants, agreements and vows:

1 Samuel 20:8 and 16-17

Therefore thou shalt deal kindly with thy servant; for thou hast brought thy servant into a covenant of the LORD with thee: notwithstanding, if there be in me iniquity, slay me thyself; for why shouldest thou bring me to thy father? So Jonathan made a covenant with the house of David, saying, Let the LORD even require it at the hand of David's enemies. And Jonathan caused David to swear again, because he loved him: for he loved him as he loved his own soul.

When David himself became king, he remembered the covenant between him and Jonathan. Saul was now dead, as were all of his sons, but David had not forgotten that covenant with Jonathan:

2 Samuel 9:6-7

> *Now when Mephibosheth, the son of Jonathan, the son of Saul, was come unto David, he fell on his face, and did reverence. And David said, Mephibosheth. And he answered, Behold thy servant! And David said unto him, Fear not: for I will surely shew thee kindness for Jonathan thy father's sake, and will restore thee all the land of Saul thy father; and thou shalt eat bread at my table continually.*

God is a covenant-keeping God. He will certainly keep His end of any contract, and with His grace being continuously extended to us, He expects us to do the same:

Deuteronomy 7:9

> *Know therefore that the Lord thy God, he is God, the faithful God, which keepeth covenant*

*and mercy with them that love him and keep
his commandments to a thousand generations.*

Our God is a God who restores His people.
Jehovah Shamma is His name, and He is always
there when we need Him.

Psalm 23:3

*He restoreth my soul: he leadeth me in the paths
of righteousness for his name's sake.*

The point I am making, again, is that soul
ties—for good and for evil—can be formed
through close friendships.

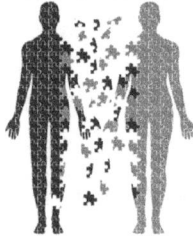

- 5 -

How to Break Unrighteous Soul Ties

Unrighteous soul ties must be broken, and here's how to do it:

- Confess each sin that was the cause of the soul tie (for instance, fornication or adultery, etc.). Repent of it and receive forgiveness.
- Collect and destroy all gifts shared during this unholy relationship, gifts like cards, flowers, rings, clothing (especially undergarments, lingerie). Anything that symbolizes the ungodly practices in this relationship must go.
- Break any vows, commitments or covenant agreements made during this

ungodly relationship and pronounce them dissolved once and for all.

- Renounce, in Jesus' name, any word curses spoken throughout this ungodly relationship. For example, "I'll never love anyone else like I love you," "I cannot live without you," "I don't want anyone but you," etc. Replace each curse with God's Word, His promises. Forgive the other person and forgive yourself for engaging in an unlawful practice (sex, the misuse of finances, etc.).

- Be honest with yourself about the guilt and the shame. Apply the atoning blood of Jesus over your life.

- Renounce the soul tie, turn from it and start walking in your deliverance.

- Open your mouth and renounce sin. Name the person or persons involved.

- Break that soul tie in Jesus' name.

- Open your mouth and declare the soul tie to be broken, including the name of the other person or persons involved.[6]

---

6. Adapted from https://www.greatbiblestudy.com/deliverance-ministry/basic-introduction-to-soul ties/

A Prayer for Deliverance from Soul Ties and a Fragmented Soul

Lord Jesus Christ, I forgive my ancestors and descendants, and I ask You to forgive and bless them. Forgive me for my many sins, and I forgive myself for sins against my body. I break all curses, hexes, vexes and demonic ties that bind me. I break all soul ties caused by witchcraft or sexual sins.

Lord Jesus, restore my fragmented soul (mind, will and emotions). Send Your angels out to recover anything that was stolen from me through this soul tie.

Lord Jesus, stir up the demons in my subconscious mind so that they can be identified and cast out.

All these things we ask in the blessed name of our Lord Jesus Christ, our Lord, Master and Savior.

We now take authority over Satan and all the forces of evil according to the whole Word of God and command that you obey it. In the name of Jesus Christ, we ask these things. Amen!

Satan, we come against all powers, principalities, evil forces in this world and spiritual wickedness in high places. We come against all demons inside or outside of anyone present, over this city, state, nation and world, in Hell or out of Hell.

The Bible says, *"Behold, I give unto you power to tread on serpents and scorpions, and over all the power of the enemy: and nothing shall by any means hurt you"* (Luke 10:19). We intend to exercise that power to set ourselves free.

Satan, we come against you by the power and blood of Jesus Christ, by the Word of God, by the name of Jesus, by the authority of the believer, in the unity of our spirits.

Satan, we tell you that we sit in heavenly places with our Christ Jesus. We are over you, your fallen angels, your demons and all forces of evil. We command you to line up in rank and file and order and come out quickly. We bind every power that you have and loose ourselves from you in the name of Jesus.

Lord Jesus, we ask that You send the gifts of the Holy Spirit as needed to minister to the needs of the people and to accomplish what

You want done here. We will be careful to give You all the glory, honor, praise and credit for everything that is said or done.

We ask all these things in the blessed name of Jesus Christ, our Lord and Master and Savior. And we take authority over Satan according to the whole Word of God.

For it's in Jesus' name we pray.
Amen!" [7]

---

7. This prayer was written by Gene B. Moody and is adapted from his *Deliverance Manual,* no copyright

Sexual Sin Demons

Learn to recognize and overpower demons of sexual sin. Some of them are:

- Masturbation	- Multiple Sex Partners
- Fantasy Lust	- Bestiality
- Oral Genital Sex	- Homosexuality
- Anal Sex (Sodomy)	- Lesbianism
- Pornography	- Perversion
- Fornication	- Reprobate Mind
- Adultery	- Molestation
- Rape	- Incest
- Spirit Whoredoms	- Idolatry
- Immorality	- Prostitution
- Incest	- Voyeurism [1]

Before going through the process of sexual sin deliverance, you should go through your home and collect any and all related paraphernalia. This would include books, magazines, sexual objects, pictures, etc. Please

1. This list is not conclusive.

destroy these items. Do not pass them down to a friend.

Acts 19:19

> *Many of them also which used curious arts brought their books together, and burned them before all men: and they counted the price of them, and found it fifty thousand pieces of silver.*

Deliverance from and the Renunciation of Sexual Sins

I renounce all sexual sin that I have been involved with in the past, including fornication, masturbation, pornography, perversion, fantasy, and adultery in the name of Jesus.

I break all curses of adultery, perversion, fornication, lust, incest, rape, molestation, illegitimacy, harlotry, and polygamy in the name of Jesus.

I command all spirits of lust and perversion to come out of my stomach, genitals, eyes, mind and mouth, hands and blood in the name of Jesus.

I present my body to the Lord as a living sacrifice (Romans 12:1).

My members are the members of Christ. I will not let them be the members of a harlot (1 Corinthians 6:15).

I release the fire of God to burn out all unclean lust from my life in the name of Jesus.

Soul Ties: An Inside Look

I break all ungodly soul ties with former lovers/sexual partners in the name of Jesus.

I cast out all spirits of loneliness that would drive me to ungodly sexual relationships in the name of Jesus.

I command all spirits of hereditary lust from my ancestors to come out in the name of Jesus.

I command all spirits of witchcraft that work with lust to leave in the name of Jesus.

I take authority over my thoughts and bind all spirits of fantasy and lustful thinking in the name of Jesus.

I cast out all marriage-breaking spirits of lust that would break covenant in the name of Jesus.

I cast out and loose myself from any spirit spouses and spirits of incubus and succubus in the name of Jesus.

I cast out all spirits of perversion, including Moabite and Ammonite spirits of lust, in the name of Jesus.

I receive the spirit of holiness in my life to walk in sexual purity in the name of Jesus (Romans 1:4).[8]

---

8. By John Eckhardt, *Prayers That Rout Demons* (Lake Mary, FL: Charisma House, 2007), used by permission

Author Contact Page

Jane P. McCoy
Broken Wings Healing Ministries International
P.O. Box 366
Carencro, Louisiana 70520

Phone: 337-356-1583

www.janeministries.org

Jane Ministries on Facebook @janeministries
Personal Facebook ID: Jane McCoy

Books by
Jane P. McCoy

Breaking Free

Free

A Manual for Finding Deliverance through Prayer and Fasting

Jane P. McCoy

One Flesh

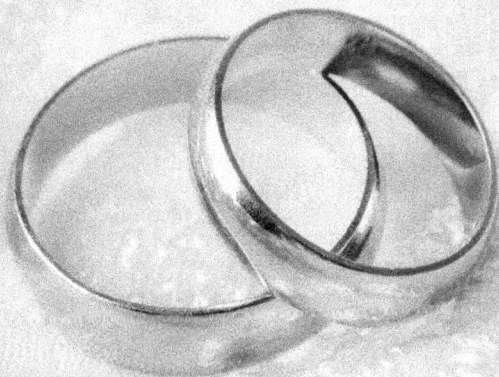

Discovering Kingdom Principles for Your Marriage

Jane P. McCoy

UNMASKING THE ROARING LION

Understanding Fear and Its Design

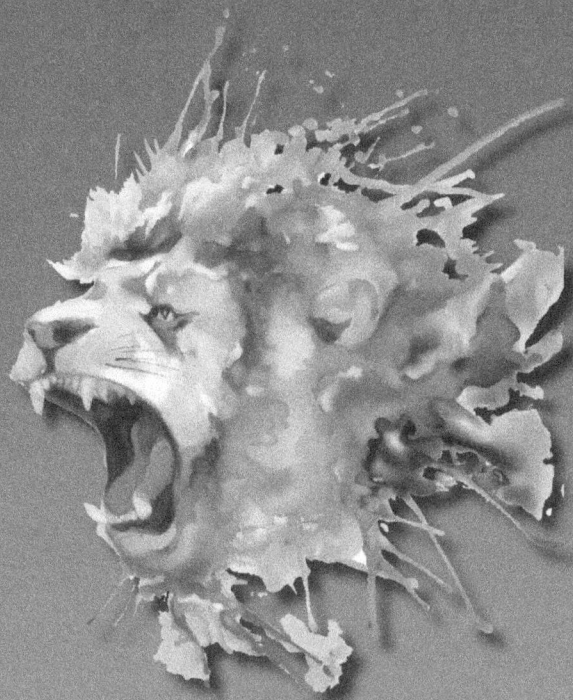

JANE P. MCCOY

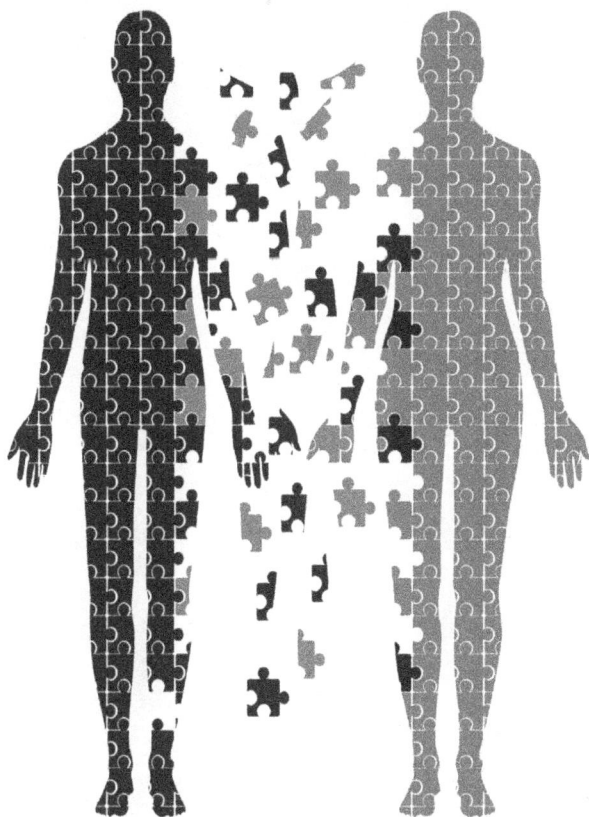

www.ingramcontent.com/pod-product-compliance
Lightning Source LLC
Chambersburg PA
CBHW031608040426
42452CB00006B/447